The Hypnotic Wisdom of Weight Loss

Steve Ashman

About the Author

Steve Ashman is a Certified Hypnotherapist, Stage Hypnotist and Master Practitioner of Neuro Linguistic Programming and works in practise in Leicestershire, England. As a therapist he specialises solely in weight management and Hypno-Band, hypnotic gastric band surgery.

In addition to therapy, Steve tours with his show 'The Hypnotic Wisdom of Weight Loss', sharing his experience in the field of weight management and how hypnosis can be used to fascinating effect to improve many aspects of your life.

Steve is contactable through his web site at:

www.ashmanhypnosis.co.uk

Dedication

This work is dedicated to my wife, Marion Ashman for her love and support, to my friends and colleagues who work tirelessly in this industry and all of my clients that have benefited from hypnosis over the years.

Copyright

Table of Contents

Chapter 1 - Our Misconceptions and Belief Systems

Chapter 2 - Achieving Balance and Changing Patterns

Chapter 3 - Planning your Future

Chapter 1 - Our Misconceptions and Belief Systems

Weight gain in our lives happens slowly. It sneaks up on us. Our shape expands until our clothes hang uncomfortably, bulging in all the wrong places. Psychologically the mind games begin creating a guilt ridden complex of views that force the highs and lows of dieting to engulf our lives, with periods of positive abstention and uncontrollable bingeing. Having experienced this phenomenon, you may question that the stability in your life has something to do with weight gain or remain with the fact that you may never be able to change the way you think.

Are we happy with how we look?

Or are we simply reacting to how our peers may perceive or talk about us?

The Hypnotic Wisdom of Weight Loss is here to dispel all the myths, to strip away existing thought patterns and play with what you believe to be real.

...and what is expected of you, I hear you ask?

Climb aboard and enjoy the ride. Let the information in this text flow over you and challenge what you've always known to be correct because quite often, all is not what it seems. You will need to apply yourself. Put into action the things you've learned and plan your future. Importantly you will need to learn to prepare your personal life for change.

Change is inevitable in all of us. Sometimes for the good and sometimes for the bad, at least the Hypnotic Wisdom of Weight Loss will allow you to make decisions that will guide you to the greater good, a better life, a happier life and a slimmer life.

Eat less and exercise more

The saying is true.   Creating a balance between what you eat and how much you exercise is ultimately the answer to consistent managed weight loss.   Those that choose to diet quickly do lose weight for a time with the risk of it returning all too quickly in times of stress and distracted will power. Whereas, few overweight people find the energy and moral fortitude to exercise while the pain in their limbs and joints continue to create a pattern of misery. The balance of exercise and nutrition is a true dichotomy and mastering both of these elements is the way forward. Achieving a natural balance of healthy nutrition and exercise promises to give you the body shape and weight you strive for. Achieving this balance comes with many, not easily apparent additional benefits, which this text will explore.

But, it's easier to say than do. Constraints on our working patterns, commitments in our private lives and a cocktail of lethargy and tiredness divert our good intentions and will power. What was once for you as a younger person, a free form lifestyle without commitment, can quickly become clouded with parental responsibility and economic worries. In a short period of time lives quickly become complex where spontaneity is replaced by set patterns that have a stark effect on our overall well-being.

Tried every weight loss program on the market?

Do you feel helpless, as if nothing will work for you?

Don't stop now, read on. The Hypnotic Wisdom of Weight Loss explores the patterns in your thoughts that create your understanding of nutritional normality, giving

you time to create effective understanding
and direction.

Stuck in a rut!

As you pass through life, you create patterns in the same way that a farmer creates furrows in a field.   The more prolonged the activity, the deeper they are. These patterns determine our outlook to life and set parameters as to what we can achieve. The saying 'stuck in a rut' is a clear analogy.   In the farmer's case, moving the tractor in a different direction requires additional power to break the cycle. In our lives, the psychological rut needs to be eradicated to allow free thinking, a lateral movement of ideas which creates the ability to think out of the box, moving you away from mainstream thought. This 'everything is possible' outlook allows us to tailor direction to suit our ambition.

Not all of us will want to achieve the lofty heights of Felix Baumgartner, parachuting out of an hot air balloon at 128,000ft or running fifteen consecutive marathons across the summer months, especially when our existence in recent years has been to vegetate on the sofa, eating exotically whilst engrossed in a Hollywood blockbuster. As a person with a history of weight issues, goals of almost any magnitude may seem clearly beyond the realms of possibility.

But, dreaming is part of the answer. When you fail to dream and accept what life throws at you, you are at the mercy of the waves. Like a game of whack-a-mole, waiting for the next disaster to draw your attention and zap your energy. Dreaming all day long may not be a productive answer to your issues of being overweight, but clarity of thought and direction certainly are.

I have no dreams, I'm happy with my lot in life!

The 2011 Great British Bake off Winner, Jo Wheatley typifies many of us in our adult years, devoted for so many years to her children, their education and nutritional welfare and a clear driven passion of the culinary art. I was pleased to see her joy as the winner of the show, humbled by the accolade as champion. Her focus may not have been planned or premeditated, but both areas of her life are outstanding achievements. The defining moment of the show is when the winner is revealed, the surprise on her face, the pride and the high that the person rides making all of the effort worthwhile.

As you take on this hypnotic journey those days will happen for you too. At first, the achievements you make may be small. A short walk here, a few pounds lost there, maybe even a small activity that you haven't done for a long time, but the pleasure principle will have been ignited. If you like what you are doing, you will want to do more. Your self esteem will increase and strangely,

you will become inspirational in others eyes –
I guarantee it.

The psychology of the yo-yo diet

Been there, done that?

"I've tried every diet on the market and they simply don't work!" is a mantra I hear all too often in the therapy room.   Dieters who crave the thin life often search out a hypnotherapist as a last ditch attempt to lose weight, after bouncing from one weight loss system to another.

So what is going on?

You might suspect a rhythmic cycle, each part of a day creating a different set of characteristics and emotions when the mind is at rest or occupied.   At one moment you can be experiencing an overwhelming optimism for life, a care free attitude, where nothing fazes you.   Then, only a few hours later, emotions will be reversed, perhaps triggered by the disappointment of the image in the mirror or the latest fashions that look better on others, than they do on you. The time you allocate to mindful distraction or relaxing solitude can have as a big an impact on calorific intake as those emotional triggers.

First of all, to have attempted a diet in the first place you have climbed to the first step. You have realised you need to do something. For some of us this feeling comes at an early stage when the weight is easily moved, for others the move from major obesity is only prompted by a traumatic family event or a visit to the doctor's surgery and the warning of death. Nothing motivates our reluctance more than to hear 'lose weight or die', a characteristic discussion that so many diabetes and heart attack sufferers hear.

Staying with the human condition for a moment, the will power required to make the change is charged with a driving force, emotion. Emotion is important, we need to get emotional. If you decide to parachute, the chasm between the leap from safety to a successful landing on the ground is a wide spectrum beginning with apprehension, moving to outright fear to complete relief. Without the emotion what would be the reward? The successful completion of achievements delivers self esteem and pride, emotions often lacking in the overweight.

Now you may have reached this stage before, will power charged by copious amounts of emotion.

Then why did you fail to lose weight and slip back?

Will power requires your attention for 365 days a year, 24 hours a day. The moment that you focus your attention away from this goal your guard is down. How many times have you been at work and told everyone you are on a diet and must be good. Colleagues around you that don't need to diet, do little to support your cause, flooding the office with sweet filled temptations, celebratory cakes and take away lunch offerings. Then comes the day when your attention has been distracted, a family crisis, issues at work, stress that consumes your thinking and you give in. The diet no longer seems important in the scheme of things. You see the diet as bolted onto your life, an unnecessary barrier that you can easily bring back into play at a better time. At that moment it has little value, some brief release from the pressures of the day is favoured and the eating begins again.

Later that day, the issues have all subsided. What was all important at lunch time, a life and death situation seems irrelevant except now the image in the mirror is still overweight, maybe now even more so. The yo-yo cycle continues, fluctuating with the seasons. In the few occasions that dieters break out and appear free from weight issues, their improvement is often associated with traumatic events, like redundancy from work, divorce or bereavement. How many times have you noticed newly single people look the best they have in years, all of a sudden they seem to strive for new goals breaking the chains of the yo-yo diet.

Don't get me wrong, I am not recommending divorce as a drastic method of weight loss. Although from this moment on, you should remove will power and guilt from your thinking. Only the doggedly determined master will power, as it requires your attention all the time and let's face it the normal individual with a complex life cannot do this. Nobody I know can forsake all other aspects of their life to motivate their will power for complete focus and control. Like I say, one emotional slip and will power is flushed away until the next burst of good intention, an emotional trap.

And where did feeling guilt and regret really get you? Nowhere.

The three emotions of guilt, shame and regret weave themselves into our physical being and make very little positive difference. In fact, the effects of these emotions are completely negative and out balance any conscious efforts we make to refine or improve our lives. These emotions alone are enough for you to want to choose more food as a comfort.   Let's take one example.   Your month has been successful in your eyes. You have planned and shopped for healthy food, taken a bus and exercise to work where you would have normally driven, started a new hobby and exercised at the weekend. On Monday evening you are presented with an evening meal at a restaurant you hadn't planned for. A family event that couldn't be avoided and you've eaten the meal slowly and enjoyed it. Now, this situation could so easily have turned sour with guilt and regret playing their part, but without them a positive outcome is so much more common. You see without guilt you can only look forward. Without guilt, you can fill the gap with an entirely more appropriate emotion. Just think what would happen, if you substituted guilt with determination or any other positive feeling? I am not saying make a life where you break rules and its OK, what I am saying is that situations will arise seemingly out of your control, stay positive.

By layering positive emotions and moving forward we build our self esteem, an important part of weight loss and finding balance. Self esteem changes our view point and allows us to re-evaluate what is important in the wider concept of our lives. Self esteem is a global emotion that spills out into every aspect of what you do and what you think. Build your self esteem first. Play with all of your positive emotions, cultivate them and enjoy the ride. With every goal you achieve take the opportunity to feel great about you, the person. Discover the bigger picture. The small matter of weight management will soon become an integrated part of your life, a collection of strategies and decisions that support your aims, no longer isolated.

The drive for health and well-being

Let's start at the beginning, why do you want to lose weight?

Is this question really so simple to answer?

Defining the why is important. Why? Like all goals if you aren't specific, if you don't set a destination, if you aren't clear as to the purpose of the task or goal how will you know if you have succeeded?

For example; 'I am going to lose 2 stones in weight so that I no longer need that knee operation', is a clearly defined statement of intention and goal. However, 'I want to lose weight because my partner wants me to look slimmer', lacks either of those things. Knowing exactly what you want out of life is the most important aspect of the weight loss battle. Be sure you know how much you want to weigh, how good you will feel and the exact date you are going to be there. Or how will you know you are successful? It is also important to understand the why, the emotional driver that makes this change appropriate and possible.

The obvious drivers for change are health, the influence of close family and those looking to have more energy and feel fitter in all aspects of their lives. This list, of course is not exhaustive. In terms of health, a medical scare may be all that is needed to motivate a person to look after their overall lifestyle. The scare may not be limited to the individual, but immediate family members or close friends where an emotional link exists. The very thought of suffering or going through the same pain or worry will often act as enough leverage to make important change happen.

Probably the largest effect on a person's life is the values and beliefs that originate from those closest to them.   The social connection between immediate family members may unknowingly create additional issues in terms of weight loss, even though the support created by this network of people is built on good intention.   Making and instigating changes in life may sit uncomfortably with others who are happy with their lot in life. Rarely are these feelings generated by malice or envy.   So often they simply want to protect a spouse or dependant from disappointment, values generated and reinforced by their own life experiences.

In the same way as a parent, bringing children into the world is a lifetime commitment. You will always put the needs of your children first, but this should not put your life on hold in the meantime. Parenthood is exactly the same as any other goal you strive to achieve. Balanced nutrition will become part of your overall plan moving forward.

Are you looking for support from your nearest and dearest?

Support can be a hurdle. Those around you will not necessarily understand your motivations. By introducing changes a little at a time you will give everyone in your support network the chance to get on board. Many of you may have already realised that shouting the word diet runs the risk of your efforts being ignored or at worst ridiculed with timely reminders of previous episodes.

If you are a person with a child centric lifestyle, where your world revolves around their needs and activities, you'll realise that your children's belief systems are created by their parent's example. How can you not be acting responsibly by being clear about nutrition and a healthy lifestyle? The planning phase of this book will prove a big hit with children and adults alike. Believe it or not, creating bright, happy memories is a way of associating positive motivation, exercise and perfect nutrition.

Have you ever sat next to someone that has a got the bug?

Perhaps you've met the super fit athlete, footballer or gym junky that seem to radiate happiness and enthusiasm. They look fabulous in their clothes and maybe you admire them for their seemingly never ending achievements and popularity or maybe you are one of those people that just feel uncomfortable by their presence. The truth is if you are listening to their protestations, boasts or words of encouragement from a place of lethargy you won't get the message. Until you find your own motivations and achieve things that are emotionally attached to your life, then you may still feel resentment towards the world and its people that seem to effortlessly evolve. Yet when the bug takes hold of you, ultimately you will achieve your desired weight and opportunities in life begin to expand way beyond your wildest dreams. Being fit, healthy and energetic is a drug with a massive positive effect. You can do so much more and feel so much better, more of the time and more people will want to be around you.

And finally, there are those that want to live an exceptional life. What does that mean, exceptional life?

It means you won't accept what life throws at you, you want to stretch your understanding, visit more places, know more things, create lasting memories that no one can take away and smile uncontrollably. These people are not overweight. The TV dinner does not beckon them. Food is secondary in their lives because they don't focus on it and if they want a giant burger, a side and massive fries they can have it After all, with all of the movement they are doing and the energy they are emitting few would argue minute meals are really needed. It is at this point that the plot unfolds. This book is going to take you through the many aspects of food, but essentially it is more to do with you and how you want to be and live and from this platform you will have the body you have always craved.

Getting the best nutrition

There are millions of books on the market that will highlight the calorific content of every food group, making recommendations as to your consumption by the hour and the day. I don't want you to start with this. You are intelligent. You have tried every diet going and I'm sure you know what the no-no products are. Pork dripping sandwiches and chips for every meal are not the way forward, I'm sure you already agree. I can hear you say, but I need to be told what to eat. To be sure I need calorific values, points per item or a list of healthy items and importantly, details of the specific magic element which is going to make me thin. Clearly cabbage has had a profound impact on all of our lives.

The point is, this is not a diet. This is a change to your long term association to food. In the past, the week before your diet you may have been enjoying a cooked meal each evening, accompanied by wine, occasional take-aways and hot chocolate drinks with all of the marsh mallow trimmings. Then week one of the diet you are reduced to food in multiple shades of green, long periods of feeling hungry and other healthy options. Of course, in week one your will power is high, but by the first weekend all too many of us have fallen off the wagon and returned to old habits which we know are bad for us. When we return to our old foods, we've normally missed the taste so bad that we eat even more and the yo-yo diet is set in motion. Add lashings of guilt and life can seem pretty miserable.

How does our mind process the relationship with food?

Take for example, a bar of chocolate sitting in the fridge. At night-time when the hustle and bustle of the day has alleviated, you've put the kids to bed and finally, there's me time. On a diet you open the fridge door and see the chocolate, you consciously close the door aware that you are on a diet and return to the TV to relax. Although you never truly relax, your conscious and subconscious minds remain on a heightened state now distracted from normal thought in anticipation of chocolate. By the end of the next TV commercial you are back in the kitchen, perusing, roaming and attempting to fight the inevitable. Then whoosh, the wrapper is off and the whole thing is devoured and if you're honest with yourself you really haven't enjoyed it. Oops and then guilt, the yo-yo effect is back in action.

A Hypno-Band client of the practise explained she had previously fought her diet cycle by starving herself for the two days before the weekly weigh in at the diet club and rewarded her efforts with chips on the way home if a new target had been achieved. She was understandably embarrassed until I laughed at the ludicrous situation. Don't get me wrong weight loss clubs are not bad, they offer cooking skills and information about food which are valuable tools in creating a new life. But failing to turn up at the class to avoid the shame because you know your weight has increased by a few extra pounds does little for your self esteem. Remember banish guilt, regret and shame. These are all negative emotions that have no positive effect on your life.

Now let's cover the basics of good nutrition.   We all need food to live. We all love food. Few people can argue those facts.

1.   Learn to be Creative

For the majority of us our food diaries are a limiting factor in healthy nutrition. When considering a change to our dietary habits a good place to start is to create a daily record of what we eat. For most of us a core selection of ten or so recipes is all we ever cook. We supplement this minor menu with precooked additives such as microwave meals, take-aways, drive through dinners and meals at restaurants and pubs. I do appreciate that there are some Masterchef stars out there with their Pampered Chef range of kitchen equipment and delicatessen habits that make the effort to try something new and host successful dinner parties, but for most of us this is not the case. How can there be so many cooking programmes on the TV churning out recipe after recipe which we are sure we would enjoy and yet we fail to experience in our own homes. Imagine for a moment, researching, preparing and creating one new exciting meal every month. Not only would you excite your taste buds and feel a sense of achievement, within a year your stock recipe count would have increased to over twenty adding more variety to your life.

How much time would it take?

Ten minutes on the internet to find something that is within your realms of ability, adding the ingredients to your existing shopping list and another thirty minutes to cook it. Am I wrong or couldn't even busy people do that, so why don't we do it? The simple answer is preparation. When we look at our capabilities in business as an example, Isn't it strange that we all work around tight process and structure. It seems our careers are automatically progressive as we strive for the lofty heights of the next pay grade, perhaps supervisor or manager or even business owner. If we applied this approach and skills in our personal life would we be more successful? The business the saying is true, spend twenty per cent of your time in preparation and reap the rewards.

Is it really important to be more creative?

Who really needs five hundred recipes on standby?

The number of recipes is not important, variety is. By limiting our range of nutritious options we are essentially imprisoning our bodies, accepting the pathway or ruts that we have previously laid down. With only ten recipes in our food arsenal we have a fortnightly pattern that gets replenished at the supermarket without much thought at all. The trolley fills with the usual value. 25% alcohol, 10% toiletries, 30% on the staple food, 20% on meat and the rest on the fripperies, biscuits, cheese, DVD's or anything that is persuaded into the weekly shop.

Even the claims from the head of household protesting the need for vital purchases can turn a simple trip to the shops into a gluten fest, where additional items make their way into an already abundant larder.   It seems there will always be times deemed special occasion that warrant the additional push for Chinese takeaway or pizza, although the word special is diminished by the regularity of our purchases. As a nation of individuals who can purchase the ingredients for a Christmas dinner as part of their weekly shop, the element of grand banquet dining and special occasion have drifted into history. Eating has become a comfort regime and all of the magic has gone.

What is the trigger in your life that warrants the purchase of take-away food over your own?

Do the best parts of your culinary repertoire really not compare to the wizardry skills of the other external vendor?

2. Eat smaller amounts of better quality

Do our taste buds crave poor quality food, that if we are honest with ourselves has little or no flavour or do we simply bulk up our intake to satisfy our craving. Most diets are a project aimed at replacing the foods we eat with healthy alternatives. It's not uncommon for bread to be substituted for rye biscuits, red meat for chicken or a vegetarian soya derivative and full fat dairy products for skimmed varieties. I am not about to say any of these products are bad for you, in fact many of them will enhance the recipe options we have previously highlighted.   There is nothing wrong with being aware of the products you use the most and switching them in an aim to reduce fat and lower cholesterol.

The interpersonal relationship we have with our families will also influence this decision. You may have generated enough will power to begin a diet, but when you begin making the substitutions you could be walking into a barrage of abuse or complaining. It is so easy for family mealtimes to turn into a disjointed array of different recipes and separate requirements all served in a staggered seating plan.

In my own family, satisfying the needs of younger children with the more complex appetites of the mature adults continues to be a challenge and it can only help that you are creative, offering a wider range of recipes. Some of your creations will be rejected whilst others become firm regular favourites.   Of course, this has the added benefits of spending at least one meal a day at the table with the whole family, culturally something that is almost lost in modern society.

Make a list of your favourite foods, what are they?

Beef Stew, Spaghetti Bolognese, Sweet and Sour Pork, Chicken Kiev, Fish and Chips, Soup. Whatever your list is, it will have a similar feel to the one above, a blend of staple food groups first experienced in childhood with a scattering of favourite tastes developed over many years of adult development.   Now, what would happen if you bought lean mince instead of the basic fatty version, made your own fresh soup instead of packet dried or tinned, use fresh chicken instead of frozen? You may feel that purchases of this type will have a detrimental effect on the cost of your weekly shop or that continually buying fresh produce will have an impact on the amount of shopping trips you need or that good quality will have little or no impact on your overall weight. In all of these things you would be wrong.

If you appreciate quality, you are training your palate to taste and accept the difference in foods. As time passes by your unconscious mind will begin to reject the taste of lesser quality derivatives. Right now if you are overweight you have less distinction, all food is eaten almost regardless of taste. You have decided what you do and don't like, creating a set of parameters in which your mind follows without question. Without some prior recipe planning a trip to the supermarket will include a biased predefined route around likable isles, whilst your eyesight merrily deletes all manner of possible alternatives. Have you ever taken the time to look at the shelves more closely? Perhaps one single ingredient you've never considered before may just spark a little imagination, an open door to a new recipe or taste experience. The majority of what you buy isn't special, just a list of regular items. They don't stick out in your mind as being exceptional and they do little to enthuse you. This is why you treat yourselves to Chinese Take-aways, Fillet Steak in a restaurant and Curries. It is so easy to use a social or stressful situation to step away from the kitchen. Take-aways and treats are in such abundance in our lives that they are no longer special and remain even more detrimental to health. The cost of one meal out or a takeaway will quickly erase the additional cost of the quality option.

Of course, we need to consider our approach to food preparation. Every purchase doesn't have to be highest grade if cooked correctly. In terms of meat, lesser quality cuts, when cooked properly can be an economic and taste triumph – be creative.

3. Eat it slowly

Appreciation is the name of the game. Now that we have quality produce, why would we eat it quickly?   If we eat quickly the transit of food bypasses our taste buds with the resulting effect that we confiscate whatever satisfaction we would have gleamed in terms of taste. By supplying our stomachs with a continuous train of material we overwhelm our feeling of being full and move directly to the bloated stage, where the first emotions generated are regret, guilt and remorse. Cars and petrol stations have a lot to answer for when it comes to controlling weight. Leaving work late, feeling hungry and the temptations of the special offer at point of sale are always tempting. In a similar vein, doing your local shop at a supermarket whilst hungry will heighten your awareness of high sugar, high fat products which satiate our short term hunger.

I recently met a person who is having weight management issues, on arrival a large chocolate wrapper flew away in the wind as the car door opened. Not the standard size bar, but the bumper one, a delicacy even the most ardent chocolate lover would find difficult to eat in one sitting.

Now here's something to try, take a snickers or similar multi-flavoured chocolate bar. Take a few moments before you tuck in to read everything on the wrapper, every word, character and image. Reading the label may not be exciting or give you any useful information at all. It merely allows you to begin the long road of appreciation in the things you eat.   Food labels and packaging are important though, check out the e numbers, nutritional information and ingredients list on everything you buy, take an interest and become aware. Now remove the wrapper and take a look at the bar. What is the underside like? Imagine how the pattern on the underside was created by the machinery in the factory. Then look at the top of the bar and view the waves and ripples, could these have been created by pouring cooled liquid chocolate whilst the item is in motion on a conveyor belt or is air cooling used? You may never know. Processed foods are a marvel of technology, but as you decide to become more creative in your own cooking having an understanding of preparation techniques will help your food creations come alive. Looking at the wrapper and markings on the bar, do either of these things matter when you eat chocolate? Probably not. But what is important is that, you have slowed the process of digestion. By making this a slow and specific operation you have made this purchase of chocolate special. In reality, if you purchase a bar of chocolate at a service station while buying petrol you will have consumed the entire thing in less than a minute whilst driving and listening to the radio, without really enjoying it.

Now, bite a one centimetre chunk from the end of the bar, but do not bite. Push the piece between your tongue and the roof of your mouth and allow the bar to begin to melt all on its own. What taste sensation are you getting? Is it melting chocolate first or the caramel?   Savour the taste, really enjoy it. Don't do anything else. Don't watch the TV, work, simply enjoy this important moment. It may take a whole minute for the finely chopped peanuts to reach your palate and for the final coating to fade. Then cleanse your palate with water removing the last remnants of taste and repeat the process.

By making this process special you are finally enjoying the product that you have purchased. In the past, the purchase of this item would have been driven by a subconscious feeling to alleviate hunger even though an evening meal had been planned shortly afterwards.   Here's a fascinating realisation. In the past, the whole bar would have been devoured in less than the time you have just taken to remove the wrapper with little or no taste appreciation.   If you continue to eat this bar of chocolate slowly, how far will you get before the taste is actually just a little bit sickly to continue?   If our taste buds identify a sickly feeling we have the option as people to stop eating. Most of us never take this option, but at least the sensation to stop eating is being realised. This is exactly the same sensation that we want when our stomachs are full.   One of the problems of being overweight is that the food moves so quickly into the stomach that your entire plate has been devoured before your brain gets the message.   The answer is slow down.

Christmas dinner or thanksgiving is a time when you always get that unsavoury feeling of being full, three or four full courses of food plus the addition of pre-course snacks and copious alcohol. Are these really the meals that we enjoy the most or are we more satisfied when we're left wanting more? For most of us, indulging in a fine restaurant is rare occurrence where we expect to be served finely executed and presented offerings. You eat each course slowly, not only enjoying the delicate taste of each component presented by a craftsman of the art of culinary delight, but you enjoy the ambience and company of the person you eat with. The often exorbitant prices dictate how you enjoy the meal. It is special after all and normally linked with a birthday or anniversary. If you can bring this feeling of special occasion to all meal times and eat small amounts of good quality, you are well on the way to the appreciation it deserves.

4. Make meal time special

The TV dinner is the destroyer of all things social. After a long day at the office we all begin to unwind, a levelling process that brings us all down from the fury of travel and unpredictable workloads. For many of us, coming home to a cooked meal is the norm, whilst for others the coordination, planning and preparation of food is an event of multi-tasking enormity.   For you to balance a discussion with a loved one, catch up with the latest network news, eat to satiate hunger and afford enough time to allow our brains to choose a lower gear is no mean feat.   Have you noticed how the added distraction of the TV in the background kills all normal forms of communication? How often have you been berated by your partner for not actively listening to the detail of their conversation whilst your brain is in the transition to relaxation?

A conscious mind is juggling numerous bits of information until overload is achieved and the discussion between man and wife no longer has room to operate. Our conscious thinking can handle between five and nine pieces of information at anytime, any more than that and you simply can't process any more information and take any more in.

In later chapters we'll discuss planning and the benefits of preparing your meal times properly, but now the evening meal should be seen as sacred. Sit at the table with the TV off – you can always record or pause the news and watch it later. Prepare the table and sit down with your partner if you can and be prepared to give over fifteen minutes of your time to discuss the day. With no other distraction the time will become a valuable way to communicate.

But, what has this got to do with losing weight?

Nothing, directly. You won't get slim by sitting at the table and talking, but you will begin to nurture a different association to food. Serve the meal in the most attractive way you can. You may not be Jamie Oliver, Michel Roux or Gordon Ramsey, but you will begin to add culinary flair to meal times. Proceed slowly, take a mouthful and put your knife and fork down while you chew and digest. Continue to converse with your partner with your mouth empty, before taking the next mouthful.   Others at the table may eat at a rapid speed with little or no understanding or appreciation of what you are doing. Notice how much you consume in the same amount of time. The food will taste differently. Some of your favourite dishes may actually surprise you and contain flavours that may just not be palatable in large amounts. You won't change your perceptions of food overnight. You simply can't go from large amounts to almost no food in a day, that would be dieting.

With each meal, you are beginning the process of brain training. Every little change, every little suggestion you make that your unconscious mind sees as good for your health is accepted and acted upon.   By giving our meal times focus, putting them in the spot light and making them special, we begin to turn off the elements detrimental to our nutritional targets. By eating snacks on the fly, grabbing anything that comes to hand and even relishing poor quality all become secondary issues.   Now here's the weird thing I am going to tell you, if you really fancy something extra, outside of specified meal times have it. Don't hold back. I have to keep saying this. This program is not a diet. At this stage we are simply beginning the process of changing direction, one bit at a time. Each tiny change will be so small in the grand scheme of your life that you won't even realise its happened.   Let's face it, there will be things in your life that are really, really difficult to change.   If I asked you to tell me why you are overweight I bet you could give me the definitive reason. It may be snacking at lunchtimes, an abundance of chocolate, an addiction to coca cola or reliance on alcohol to relax. At this juncture in the process continue to enjoy these things.   I will guarantee that by the time you have implemented the Hypnotic Wisdom of Weight Loss in your life these items will be inconsequential and require no further thought.

Making meal times special will need some further thought. When we begin to look at planning our meals in later chapters of this book, these events will become so special that you will want to do it properly. The food will be high quality, will stand out in terms of an event and will soon be preferable to any form of take-away or processed product.

5. Planning

The trip to the supermarket is rarely planned. At best our weekly shop relies on a poorly formatted list of essentials with the remains of our purchases being made on the value proposition of the product and our desire at the time.   Again step back. Look at the whole process.

Is this how a successful restaurant would be run?

Well if the restaurant's kitchen relied on frozen food, warmed in a microwave, bulk buying of the staple goods, rice, potatoes and pasta and your menu was fixed from one month to the next with little or no variation, it is unlikely it would still be in business never mind successful. When you are looking to eat out your focus should be on quality, the type of place that takes into account product seasonality, preparing meals that are evocative, innovative and nutritious.   If you keep this train of thought in mind ask yourself, how many restaurants now live up to your very high standards?

Run your life like it's a successful business. Take some of your time each week to plan and careful execution will bring immediate results. This is the key to your success. It doesn't take long and just needs a little discipline for this to happen.

It isn't hard to find evidence to support this. Your food cupboards at home like everyone else's will contain items that have been there for years. In our home recently, a myriad of old spice jars were guided surreptitiously to the refuse bin as the contents clearly, after years of degradation hugged each glass jar in ever increasing solidity. As a couple we had always felt that these would one day become useful, a distant objective that without planning would ever materialise. It is so useful to be inspired and motivated by TV food programmes, recommendations by friends and everyday situations, it's the planning and execution that matters and is the element that lets the process down. If on your next trip to the supermarket you purchase Arborio rice simply because you ate satisfying paella on holiday in Spain, you will fall fowl of another ingredient that will make a solitary existence on your shelves. Our homes are often so crammed with ingredients that it is impossible to see what we do have in stock and end up buying the same item again and again, even though we don't need it. Larders and store rooms do not have the monopoly on over storage, deep freezers and fridge compartments are also culprits. In this realm, unlabelled produce can look exactly the same as everything else when frozen. The healthy anticipation of defrosting a korma curry and discovering the contents to be the meagre pickings of homemade vegetable soup rarely satisfies anyone's appetite.   Aim to make meals with fresh produce and use the freezer as a tool to deliver value. With this in mind, many of us will still consider the economic argument of pre-packed, pre-prepared frozen food to be stronger than the obvious benefits of eating healthy nutritious food.

How can you really establish the economic facts behind your nutrition unless you consider all aspects of your spending?

We may all be aware of the cost of our weekly shop and subsequent daily top ups of fresh bread, milk and minor purchases, but can we really account for the stock pile of ingredients in our larders and frozen meals.

Spread across multiple years, at what point in our calculation are these included?

Purposeful planning will ensure that the trend of over usage and bulk buying is eradicated and monthly expenses will be kept to a minimum.

Building a stock list

Before making a list of what to buy for the next round of recipes we need to have an accurate representation of what ingredients we already have. First of all divide an A4 page into six sections. Label those sections, dairy, frozen, tinned, dried, vegetables and meat. Then conduct a stock take and while you do, arrange the shelves so you see the items clearly. Rotate fresh goods and keep a note of items and their sell by dates.

Doesn't sound difficult or much like planning does it?

Now unless you find things which are beyond their sell by date, don't throw them out. Diet shows on the TV often start their own particular weight less system by emptying the freezer and pantries of all fattening produce from the unsuspecting dieter. A few complain whilst others have abject horror written all over their faces. In real life no one could afford such waste, but the hapless viewer goes along with the charade knowing that all costs are covered by exorbitant television fees. In your home environment this could mean hundreds of pounds of edible food being unceremoniously ejected into your wheelie bin.   Don't do this. Remember this is not a diet and few people can afford to dump food. The creation of the stock list is to make you aware of where you can start to use your imagination.

Be an auditor. Take a note of what already resides in your cupboards. Items bought with good intentions as you browsed the super market some months ago, but never really finding the time to use. In my cupboards you would find Arborio rice, famed ingredient of risotto, five or six types of pasta all shapes, an assortment of frozen food both shop bought and left over's, rotting vegetables and salad that would invariably be thrown out, a shelf of small seasonings and spices with the obligatory sprouting garlic well past its sell by date and not one jar of lemon curd but two! In a business who in their right mind would buy stock and put it on the shelf without an order. Leaving food aside for a moment, if you ran a technology style business most of the items would go out of date within a few weeks making obsolete technology hard to shift.   You wouldn't stock your shelves with the old models would you, where's the sense in that?

With the stock list in hand you have a list of core ingredients at your disposal.   From this list you can immediately begin to create a menu of meals without returning to the supermarket for additional supplies. Look for the patterns of produce. From what we already know, a lot of the ingredients will substantiate your core of ten or so recipes that you regularly eat which is fine for the moment. We can now begin to play and use our imaginations using the remaining items in the list. In most households you'll be amazed to find at least a fortnight of evening meals, even though your next trip to the shops is already planned.

This has two immediate effects. The first, it begins to reduce your stock holding of ingredients to a manageable level. Less money will have been spent on items that take up space and in the main remain in the larder.   Secondly, by removing the need to go to the shops you are less inclined to replenish your stores with biscuits, cakes and other fripperies. If they aren't in your home, how can you be tempted to eat them?

The power of imagination

To go from a core set of recipes to a completely avant-garde menu overnight isn't going to happen. Start small and slowly introduce something new. Start by looking at items with a sell by date. Of course, we could freeze many of these items nearing expiry, but let's elevate the word fresh in our awareness to begin with. At this point you need to dream. Yes, waste a few minutes, break out of the zone which compels you to make the same old stuff. The internet, food programmes or cookery books are perfect for this. It doesn't matter what ingredient you have on the list, whether it's an obscure ingredient or more mainstream component, either search in the index of the book or enter it in your internet browser.

How many recipes are there for chicken, Arborio rice and pasta shapes?

I am asking you to be adventurous by choosing recipes that challenge your eating habits and appeal to your imagination. These recipes will be a simple move for anyone that is skilled in the kitchen, however if you are new to the world of culinary creation look for simple recipes at first. Ones that play with the flavours you and your family will enjoy. Avoid being too ambitious, moving too quickly from the simple to the complex overnight may sometimes backfire and fail to have the desired out come. As I said before you can quickly add a couple of satisfying dishes to your repertoire. When it comes to planning your food diaries remember, your home is not the Ritz and you won't need a full blown recipe every night. The cookery workload should not treble. In fact with planning, the time needed should in fact reduce.

Varying your nutritional menu

What does varied mean?

There is nothing wrong with a roast dinner with all the trimmings, but not every night. Adopting a successful planning procedure will assign the correct meal to the right meal time. For instance, you may prioritise the importance of a family get together and suitable meal on a Sunday, whereas other days throughout the week may call for lighter options which can be prepared quickly. You won't need to devour enormous amounts of food if your free time is allocated to the pursuit of fitness, swimming, sport or dancing, these can all be part of the changes you allow yourself to make. I still haven't mentioned reducing the amount you eat yet, have I?

By beginning to make small changes, such as auditing your cupboards, making a plan and adding a small amount of exercise to each day you are already on the way. Of course, if you were on a diet you would be engrossed in weighing yourself each morning and with each tiny piece of cheese you eat, a self generated guilt trip would emerge. There is no need for you to do this. For the moment concentrate on planning.   Get in the habit of allocating a few minutes each week to sit and think. The thought you give to planning will guide your thinking, taking your actions in a new direction. This new found direction is not based on starvation or holding back on certain specific items and you are enjoying the process.   The more you enjoy what you are doing the more you will continue. This is the pleasure and pain principle, if we enjoy something it is easy to find yourself wanting to do it more, but if you feel pain such as overdoing exercise your subconscious mind will quickly adapt to protect you and remove all semblance of will power.

As you research, varied and exciting food groups will spread vicariously through your arsenal of recipes.   If your weekly intake consisted of a large roast Sunday lunch, a take away at the weekend and an assortment of shallow and deep fried foods mid week with minor planning you will already be ahead. Replacing just one of those unhealthy options with a scintillating stir fry or vegetarian bake means that $1/7^{th}$ of the week has already been altered and you've hardly noticed the difference. Focussing on recipes that your whole family will enjoy, are easy to prepare and nutritious and will become part of you with some triumphs and disasters. Before long you will find it almost impossible to return whole heartedly to what you ate before.

As you explore new recipes develop an eye for greener ingredients. The fruit and vegetables on offer at your average supermarket are varied and can be used as a prime mealtime produce or as an accompaniment to other protein. Needless to say raw materials that are fresh are always going to be better for you than frozen. Pay attention to expiry dates, eliminating waste will keep costs down and maximise the value of your purchases. Each meal should be the main event with a careful balance of vegetables or salad. Vegetarian dishes can add an abundance of variety where previously only meat dishes were available.

Make it special - presentation

Remember, make it special. When the food is delivered to the table take time to serve it neatly and with a little flair. A plate with a lip, piled high that holds an enormous amount of food is hardly conducive to healthy nutrition. Practise, the less is more on your plate.

When you deliver your meal on a standard size white plate, can you see more of the plate than the food on it?

Make the transition from heaps of food to a small articulate design slowly. We want to make regular, small changes to our eating pattern, a method that will abate our obvious cravings. It is so easy to design a plate of food that looks attractive and remove a small element, such as one spoon of mashed potato, a scoop of pasta or reduce the mound of rice. When you set out to eat, enjoy what you have created. Don't attack the plate with gay abandon, eat it slowly, tasting every mouthful. All of these elements working together are creating new associations with food. From this moment, every meal you eat away from home will become a comparison with the quality you create.

How quickly will it be before you begin to recognise that not all restaurant meals and take-away options are as good as they should be?

There's no getting away from it, you will begin to feel disgruntled. A feeling of paying hard earned cash for poor quality food will stick in your throat. These comparisons will begin to appear everywhere. As your knowledge of food preparation swells, not only will you save money but the creation of new associations will add to your new found direction. This discerning pattern of pleasure is what we need to nurture. The more pleasure you experience, the more motivation you create allowing your subconscious thinking to continue to propel you forward.

There are many ways to gain a deeper understanding of nutrition from phone apps, to books to TV food shows. As time passes and the change in your behaviour continues to occur, you will be more inclined to choose healthy and nutritious versions over fattier or processed alternatives. It doesn't matter if you digress at any point on this journey, this is not a diet. You have changed direction and the balance of action is now firmly in the good, your weight will be reducing and the benefits of feeling lighter and fitter will add to the feeling of change.

Exercise - the pleasure and pain principle

When using will power your conscious mind is actively engaged in controlling what you eat and how you act and we now know that for will power to actually work, you need to focus on what you eat and act all of the time. This is one of the reasons why we fail. We cannot concentrate for the whole of our lives on one thing. To achieve a long term result we need to bring the subconscious mind into play. The subconscious works to keep you alive and safe. Every thought we place in the subconscious is acted upon as long as it is within the realms of possibility.

If we begin to drip feed our subconscious mind with fresh thoughts that lead towards our goals of any kind, not just weight loss we will inevitably change our own direction and create a better life. If you think back to a time when you have failed at something you will realise you had a diseased thought rattling around inside your head. A self doubt, an insecurity or a concern and the positive direction was then in conflict. Say for instance, you want to be an after dinner speaker. You know your subject well and confidence is what you are trying to instil into your performance. On one hand you are well rehearsed and can get the audience's attention, whilst on the other hand a nagging doubt possibly reinforced by others around you is telling your subconscious things like, what happens if you get a heckler? Or what if they don't find you interesting? Or what will you do if everyone just starts talking over you? Remember your subconscious mind is there to protect you and keep you safe. You may understand then, with those thoughts in your mind, the ultimate direction you are being guided in may be to give up or postpone.

I say this, because the same thing happens when you try to exercise. You take the leap of faith, your will power says today is the day, no longer am I going to be fat, I am sick of being the slow coach, the underdog. You launch without thought into a raft of exercise and you feel high. The high is important. A high which adds emotion to the event creates even more drive. Now, because most of us have been devoid of any kind exercise for quite some time we over do it. It could be something as minor as an aching shoulder muscle or a tight hamstring or more seriously sciatica caused by back trauma. The fact is no one likes pain. Our bodies are amazing and will do all they can to repair any problems we inflict on ourselves. Most exercise pain will take two to three days before easing and a further day to completely repair. For a moment let's return to the purpose of the subconscious mind to protect you and to process thoughts. The

subconscious mind picks up the message
that all is not well and acts without critical
thought to protect you, you cannot intervene.
As you sleep the unconscious mind is doing
its best to point you away from the pain.
Internal dialog runs amok, don't do that
again! Exercise is not good for you! Relax,
put your feet up! Who knows what the real
message is, all we know is eventually the
subconscious which never sleeps will
outweigh all of the hard work of the will power
still processing in your conscious awareness.

Temper your will power and allow your
subconscious mind to do what it does best.
Be clear about your intentions, take your time
and importantly, start your exercise regime
slowly. So slow in fact that you don't even
realise you have started to change. Don't
sign up for the gym membership on day one,
set an ideal date in two or three month's time.
What you do next will depend on your overall
health and BMI – body mass index. If you

take action to lose weight earlier in life chances are your joints are in a reasonable state of repair and immediate movement will do little to damage the underlying tissues. Prolonged obesity in older people needs to taken into consideration and exercise should not be undertaken without prior consultation of your GP.   Your joints if subjected to prolonged periods of obesity may have advanced forms of deterioration.   General movement around the house and to the car or local amenities can often be a painful experience. Losing small amounts of weight can have a dramatic effect and improvement on lifestyle and movement.

For the overweight with a BMI classification of obese class I, start with something simple. A walk around the block, a half mile walked on a flat service. For those obese class II and above and where discomfort is present aim for 200 metres. It doesn't seem like much does it? With a BMI of class II exercise is unlikely to be part of the normal cycle of day to day life. By applying regular movement everyday and creating routine as people we can quickly begin to get used to the effort. We are simply conditioning our muscles and joints to flow, whilst allowing the body to recuperate with short periods of rest. This means that you are not feeling excessive amounts of pain and your subconscious mind will accept this treatment as pleasure. And pleasure it soon will be! The days that you don't manage to take a walk you will soon miss as your body builds comparison.

Do the maths!

Imagine for a moment in the first 3 months you walk for 10 minutes in the morning around ½ a mile and 10 minutes later in the day, the same distance Monday to Friday. Do you realise if you do this you will walk over 250 miles a year. Incomprehensible isn't it? Even the fittest in society wouldn't set out to walk that far, but by regular activity in small amounts you are already beginning to make a difference.

So far in this text, I've said eat with more imagination, be creative and walk a little each day. There are few reading this that wouldn't be able to put these elements into immediate practise. Now, if you're reading this book for the second time and you've already done what I've asked, ask yourself this. How do you feel? It's the feeling that's important, not how much do you weigh or does my bum still look big in this? By fine tuning your brain, using your imagination and moving you are creating energy, feel good energy. Ok you haven't run a marathon yet and you haven't generated the messages of euphoria that come from crossing the finishing line, but you will have started to pick up on the conversations that the fitter in society engage. You will begin to understand why others rave about the gym, dancing and hill walking. The feel good factor is infectious.

Do I need to tell you what to do next? Do I need to give you a printed plan asking you to do squat thrusts, sit ups, muscle repetitions and the like? I could but I'm not going to do that. Use your imagination, how would you like to move? A bike-ride perhaps, a ramble, a stroll in the park - you can choose.

Now this is an important point, write it down, make a log of every piece of exercise you do. We are really recording progress, slow, steady progress. If it isn't slow and it doesn't progress then, continue to improve and change your behaviour. You may have recorded a total of 1 mile of walking in week one, increasing to 5 miles by week 5 and 10 miles by week 10, all achieved by totalling numerous, regular, small activities. You don't have to be too accurate, just fair to yourself in the estimates. Missing the odd walk isn't an issue. It's recording a clear trend that more exercise is taking place. If the trend is increasing, so will your confidence, desire and passion. Emotion is the driving force of change. People that go to the gym feel great, fair enough. But let's say they want to increase muscle and aim for a six pack or get faster times at road racing, neither will happen if they don't keep records. In weight lifting if you want to build up a certain muscle group you need to steadily increase the weight with each session, stretching the muscle which rebuilds in the rest period, this is call atrophy. Simply going to the gym and feeling good isn't enough in this case. For instance, if you record in week one, 6 sets of 6 reps each with a 10kg weight, you have in fact lifted a total of 360kg in the session. The following week to build muscle you lift 380kg in the same amount of time and so on. As the weight gets heavier you muscles may begin to fail making the final repetition impossible and by recording that effort in writing you will have an accurate record of your efforts. 380k less 1 repetition = 370kg. A lot of motivation will be gained by viewing your progress over time and the feel great factor will be an enormous secondary benefit. By failing to record your effort in writing means that you leave your workout open to conjecture and emotion.   You may feel tired, but how do you know you did enough?

Let's take another example, running. When delivered, my new shiny running machine looked impressive.   I asked a number of friends about their experiences with them and one replied 'I do about 40 minutes at a time'.   The self doubt instantly hit me. 40 minutes is an incredible amount of time to move constantly under your own steam. In past attempts at getting fit using will power I attempted runs on country roads which would hurt me even after only a few minutes. My heart and lungs gasped for air and for days afterwards the pain of stiff calves would interrupt day to day life. This is where the recording comes in. In my case, I walked on the treadmill for 6 minutes at a steady pace. Then when completely warm and comfortable I would jog for a further 10 minutes. At that time I had a bodily frame weighing seventeen stones (238lbs) and this exercise wasn't easy. Following the first few sessions I felt good about myself and didn't suffer physically for more than a couple of minutes outside of the session. By increasing the work out about once a fortnight I've steadily increased. In fact there were times when work wouldn't allow the time to exercise at the allotted time and I dropped back in terms of effort. To avoid injury you need to warm up properly and never over do it. If you miss a couple of sessions step back on your regime a little before progressing, no matter how good you feel. My exploits on the running machine and subsequently on the road have become highlights of my life. Weekly runs and workouts that produce copious amounts of positive energy, improved self esteem, keep my weight in check and have produced a series of memories that I am proud to achieve.

WARNING: That last paragraph is likely to severely turn you off!!   Until you create your own internal energy, these words will do little to motivate you. You may believe that this energy and feeling is way beyond your reach. Well I am here to tell you it is not. Get the basics right and you are already on your way to feeling amazing.

The psychology of success is derived from creating specific habits that repeated, lead you in the direction of your goals. They say do something once and it's an accident, do something twice and there's an association and do something a third time and you are already on the way to creating a habit. First of all define your convincer strategy. How many times to do you have to do something so that it becomes comfortable? So comfortable that you can repeat the operation with thinking?

When you drove a car for the first time were you like most first timers, overwhelmed by the amount of things you have to do? Pressing the pedals to produce and stop movement, adjusting direction with the steering wheel whilst constantly anticipating the action of other road users and using your mirrors before, during and after all manoeuvres . However, when you passed your driving test, how long did it take before you were totally comfortable behind the wheel, listening to the radio?

For most of us the experience of creating pleasure needs to be activated between 4 and 21 times. Whatever you set out to achieve, your unconscious mind is convinced that you can do this thing easily. At first we need to push ourselves into the zone to begin with, stretch ourselves by doing something that makes us feel uncomfortable. They say public speaking is one of the most stressful things that you can be asked to do. Yet, when you achieve the milestone of delivering a set of ideas to an audience the feeling of achievement makes it all worthwhile. Why am I telling you all this? Exercise is exactly the same. At first it's a culture shock, you aren't used to it. You don't feel comfortable and previous attempts to get fit have failed and you're not sure you enjoy it. Keep going! There is no pain and believe me the pleasure is growing. People around you will begin to sense the new you without being told. With changes in nutrition, exercise and mindset the weight will begin to fall off. Build that pleasure energy. The more pleasure energy you have the easier everything is going to be.

Don't put energy into the things you want to avoid

You now have the power and the energy to focus. Feeling good and losing weight adds a special momentum to any goals and objectives you set yourself. So when you start to plan not only your exciting food diary, but the things that you would really like to achieve in life then you will begin to realise your dreams. Be positive about everything, see the brighter side. Avoid people that nit pick your ideas or spread rumour you don't need it. You will soon discover that finding that all important direction becomes easier over time. But what happens to the difficult times, those occasions and things that you find just too hard to change. I am talking about the reasons that most of use when making excuses about not losing weight, they range from. I can't stop eating chocolate I crave it, I drink alcohol to relax, I get stressed and turn to food and my family want to eat

take-aways every Friday night. The list is
endless.

   In the early development stages of
planning you will begin to make changes to
the way you do things. The way you buy
ingredients, plan the dish and execute. The
way you decide to go out and move creating
patterns of exercise. But let's face it, you
can't plan for everything. On the night you've
decided to walk, it's raining and there is no
sense in getting soaking wet for ten minutes.
Or you have had little opportunity to get out in
the week as you have commitments with your
children.   In reality, they are danger times,
opportunities to slip backwards into old ways.
You could so easily engage your brain and
using will power stop any temptations, but
again you are in the realm of creating guilt
and shame when food is eventually eaten.
Take the pressure off. If its chocolate or a
glass of wine have it, enjoy it. No really enjoy
it. Don't feel guilty. With your new mindset

you are already adding balance to your decision making, now flex that balance muscle. The next day realise you've enjoyed and think about balance. Don't miss the walk or the run or the dance. It is so much easier to add a couple of minutes to something you enjoy like walking than it is too starve yourself and feel miserable. Step back and listen, this is not a diet, that's what you used to do. We are in the process of changing your life slowly and the truth about life is that we are all going to do things, eat things at the wrong times, in the wrong quantities – that's life. Granted we don't want to do this all the time. We are changing for the better, for the rest of our lives, so our actions have to coincide with lifestyle and our lifestyle in the long term is going to be good. We are going to feel better, be better educated, eat more nutritious food and move to build the pleasure energy, how can we not lose weight. For some, the existence of the pleasure energy is all that it takes to turn someone around. It wasn't the weight that was making them miserable it was their inability to feel good about themselves.

How has your life changed since childhood?

It's unfair to look backwards and rarely beneficial. Looking forward is a positive operation. You could though, put yourself in your own shoes when you were younger and ask yourself what was your life like then? A day in the life!

A light breakfast and then walk or bike to school, two or three miles a day. (1,000 miles a year). Charging between classrooms, physical education, football/netball practise, home for tea and out again till dark. Many of our comparisons with being busy today are more to do with stress and responsibility than actual movement. Are we in actual fact working alongside others that have similar issues, adopting their lifestyle and outlook? In most cases we have lost the ability to dream, something we would do as a child at every opportunity. You may say our imaginations have been suppressed by life experience until we accept our lot in life and the mundane activities in which we partake become the norm. It costs nothing to step outside of the box and dream. Big and small dreams are important. There is nothing wrong with thinking big, even if you know somewhere inside that your outlandish plans may not come to fruition. Who cares in the grand scheme of things, think about the journey you will embark upon, made up of smaller achievements. Shot for the stars, you may miss and hit the moon!

Excuses – I don't have time

It's hard to categorise excuses. That inner feeling that's it's easier to sit and do nothing than get up and do something. This lack of motivation sweeps across your life infecting every other positive thought. You may be sitting there finding it really hard to imagine what life will be like when you are slim and fit. It's not until you achieve a state of fitness yourself that you can stomach a slimmer's evangelising about how they lost 10 stones in 2 years, the message will always do more to turn you off than on. The facts are you will need some commitment here. Hypnosis is not a magic bullet. You can't have one session and your life is completely turned around. You are in effect a super tanker idling off shore. To turn around you need to power up enough to engage the rudder to begin the turn to create new direction and slowly you will get there. So excuses, what are yours? I am really busy at work? I used to use this one. Getting up at 5.30am in the morning to drive south somewhere around London, leaving early to miss all the traffic and then stopping for breakfast, coffee and a read of the newspaper. Before a long days work and a trip home around the M25 (Britain's biggest car park), a late finish, food at the service station and a big meal at home before sleeping on the couch. I can claim that, it did happen. The job was good the money was great and unfortunately it filled my life from one end to the other.   My goals at the time revolved around work place achievements and accolades with little in the way of personal objectives.   I wonder what would have happened if I would have adopted one or two changes? Maybe the back pain I suffered for years would not have flared and the whole experience would have been even more enjoyable. In that period of my life I didn't move, I didn't walk. I stopped in hotels and ate well and drank alcohol almost every night. I rarely switched off at night choosing to work in the room after dinner before being lured back to the bar for a late nightcap, rarely ever adopting an early night. Imagine the impact of this most days over a ten year period, balancing a weekend private life where going out for a meal with my wife and friends rarely felt like a special occasion, just another day at the office. Then came Sunday, 4 pm, the same time each week where preparation would take over and my bags would be packed for another week away. In this period of my life I learned at least one important lesson, preparation is king. You soon become worn out if you drive miles and don't execute a well drawn plan of attack. As a salesperson nothing is worse than forgetting to call a customer the day before a meeting and finding out that after a long drive the meeting is cancelled. A checklist and structure are all important.

Too busy, I haven't got time. Been there done that. The answer is that when you create a plan, look to add some balance in your schedule. Instead of sitting in the road side cafe for an hour, I'm sure I could have found a place to walk for ten minutes. I could have parked on the edge of a village or town and walked in to the centre and back. There were plenty of dry sunny days to do this. After a long drive I know my back would have appreciated this. The fatigue of driving, focussed concentration and long hours at the wheel may better have been served by exercise, perhaps a short walk at lunch at my final destination. On a dark night few of us would find getting home and waltzing around the block a pleasing option. Most of us turn on the TV, pour a glass of wine and eat food in an aid to relax, the opposite is actually true. When you do a sport that distracts the mind such as squash or football it is impossible for your conscious mind to think about anything other than the sport. This is relaxing, distressing and you do sleep better. Want to de-stress properly, add a little balance. Move. Exercise gives you a bit of time to think and then set aside half an hour to meditate with music or a hypnosis audio CD. By giving yourself that time, headaches will disappear, you'll sleep better and the next day's goals will be so much clearer. This is the ultimate promise of hypnosis – Relaxation.

Chapter 2 - Achieving Balance and Changing Patterns

What is a balanced lifestyle?

A balanced lifestyle means that you give equal priority to exercise, nutrition and mindset. For most of us this is almost impossible. When the going gets really tough and our will power is broken down, it is all too easy to slip into the things that you find easiest to do, this is human nature. By leaving decisions to the last moment you make life hard for yourself. Like what you are going to eat after work or deciding what food you are going to buy as you walk hungrily around the supermarket is leaving your will power open to fail. Its sounds impossible to comprehend, using your imagination and planning are the way to deliberate your way into a healthy routine. I've met some wonderful people in business, pure professionals that have learned the art of communication and excelled in their given subject. Their high incomes haven't been generated by chance, copious amounts of tenacity, hard work, dedication and planning have all played their part. This doesn't however always mean they have balance though. Some people work and work and rarely switch off except to enjoy the social fruits of their labour, nights out, business lunches and food on the fly. One person in particular I know is approaching what most would consider retirement, her early sixties and yet she still seems unable to find the right approach to weight control. Like others in her social circle she's tried the diets, the weight loss shakes and listened intently to those that have found a solution, but still the pounds have crept on. Now I'm not speaking about someone that's unintelligent. This is a highly successful, inspirational, business woman with all the acumen to achieve exactly what she sets out to achieve. So why hasn't permanent weight loss worked for her?

The answer is balance. Thinly veiled will power, surrounded by intellect, hiding behind a work life schedule that most of us would wince at. Take the mindset as a first place to start. When you ask a business person of this stature to tell you where they will be in five, ten or twenty year's time, they can state the figures and show you the plan without flinching. It is a clear visualisation to them. A visual mental picture that contains bright colours, sounds and importantly deep down it feels right. As a therapist you notice the signs, articulate, bright personalities that hide the real reason with such skill that it takes all your time to uncover the truth. These people are fallible like you and me, they prioritise their lives and the stuff they associate with pleasure comes first. Talking to new people is second nature. Even standing in front of an audience of hundreds which would scare most of the population of the civilised world, extolling the virtues of a value proposition, they find easy. If they, like you had balance in their lives exercise would be included in the plan and executed perfectly. I'm sure she'll read this book and I'm sure my words on page will have far more impact than a one to one in person. The fact is, there's no point being rich if your days are marred by pain or you can't travel to enjoy the spoils of your labours. If you are finding it less than easy to get around now and your weight is steadily increasing, how long will it be before you are immobile, before your knees and joints are so painful that your only movement is from the house to the car? Few of us can be this direct with a friend, but what we are actually saying makes sense. What's the point of building a business and becoming so successful if you're not around to enjoy it? With heart disease, diabetes and a hundred other problems exacerbated by being overweight why would you carry on?

The answer is balance, I can't stress this enough. Successful business people have a certain positivity that draws you in. Winning is an incredible aphrodisiac to life that it doesn't matter what approach you take to losing weight it will work. Quite simply if you generate so much pleasure energy and associate it to massive success then it's easy to lose weight. Business people have the skills. They simply need to apply those skills to the whole of their life not just the interesting part. So what do business people do as a matter of course? They set goals and plan. Importantly, they look beyond what is reasonably achievable and set goals which are incredible and then they sit down and find ways to move towards the goal. Remember when you present a positive thought to your unconscious mind, that is within the realms of possibility it is instantly actioned without question. You may take a wrong turn along the way, but overall you are moving towards that goal. Importantly, write down what you want and review it regularly.

What advice can I give the overweight business person?

Add to the top of your plan (not a secondary thought, a primary one), I am going to be fit, I am going to get people to notice my achievement, my specific weight (by this date) is going be (write it down). Be specific include the dates, the times and any important milestone along the way, big birthdays, anniversaries, holidays, anything where you can associate looking and feeling great. The promise I make is that you will have even more energy to put into your business and will feel better every day of your life.

How does the mind work?

The way the mind works is subjective in nature. The description I offer is my way of explaining something that is extremely complex. My few words will provide a base line for understanding and importantly, preparation. Other hypnotists may describe this process in other ways and all explanations may or may not be correct. The workings of the mind are like no other organ of the body. We know that we can change our minds and apply strategies to make it happen, however X-Ray machines have yet to be invented that highlight the exact process. We cannot dissect the mind in the same way that we can the heart. All that we know is that the mind is a complex process that the body needs to survive.

The mind is separated into two operating zones, the conscious and subconscious mind, sometimes called the unconscious or other than conscious. The conscious mind is like your computers RAM memory and works in real time allowing you to handle around nine actions at any time. For instance, if you are concentrating on operating something new like a mechanical digger you may well have to operate and be aware of more than one thing at a time, such as the pedals, the steering yoke, the dashboard lights, the evenness of the ground outside, etc. Whereas, the subconscious mind akin to your computer's hard drive is the storehouse of your memories holding over two million bits of information at any one time. In our example I mentioned the word new mechanical digger, as opposed to say a car, an item most of us are more familiar with.   As we become competent some actions are conducted from the subconscious mind and happen without much thought at all. Now that you've been driving for twenty years do you consciously change gear? Probably not, your conscious mind is free to work on other more important aspects such as using a mobile phone and having a conversation. (Neither of these should be conducted while the car is moving). Both zones of the mind work in harmony, with the subconscious responsible for constantly looking after your well being by regulating the heart, the lungs and the bodies organs with the conscious mind helping you to move from one place to the other, directing your legs, knees and feet.

We are a sceptical lot. Ideas are fired at us all day long and we make decisions that we feel consciously are right for our progress. The aspirations of a double glazing sales person might turn us off with a telephone call out of the blue, but will become interesting if our awareness has already been primed by need or desire. Say for instance, torrential rain had recently flooded through a broken window or one of your best friends had recently upgraded to the latest windows and doors, this influence will have broken down your critical thinking. Critical thinking is an operation that the conscious mind presents in all up front communications to directly filter ideas that others present to us. The subconscious mind in comparison has no such filtering. We can also deduce that our subconscious minds hold onto to some thoughts which hold us back from doing what's right or important. These limiting beliefs can be created early on in our lives, stored in the subconscious and recalled as situations arise. Say a child is bitten by a dog when young, that child may hold onto that fear denying them of the happiness a pet may bring.   Limiting beliefs are cognitive patterns, essentially lies we tell ourselves that are held so deeply within our subconscious that we fail to see the bigger picture and are unable to evaluate the effect they have upon us. If you take a child to a supermarket, at the checkout they seem to have the ability to continue to ask for sweets without any guilt or shame attached and invariably, win the deal, get what they want. Why is it as adults we seem to lose this ability which would be so useful in everyday business. These cognitive patterns of appropriate behaviour are formed in our minds and dictate our direction and the way we behave. By understanding how the mind works you can break these cognitive maps and get them to work for you and your weight loss goals.

The subconscious mind has no critical thinking. It simply accepts what you present to it and it goes with the idea. Successful people have positive, well thought out pictures in their minds, visualisations of their goals and where they want to be. What holds the unsuccessful back? If you present your unconscious mind with a mixture of ideas, some good, some bad, you may create more stress than achievement. Remember, the pleasure and pain principle? Build up slowly, adding exercise a little bit at a time, so that all you feel is pleasure. As you sleep at night the subconscious mind takes over and continues to look for answers, well if all of your answers, the goals, the pictures, the wants, the needs are positive expressions, how can you not succeed? If nothing else transpires you will have had a whole lot better life with reduced stress. Just imagine the possibilities.

Don't make weight your primary focus. If all you focus on in your life is your job, your family who you need to clothe and protect and your weight you are setting yourself up for a fall. Whatever you decide to set your sights on you can achieve and I can guarantee that your weight will always benefit. If you book a night class into your already busy schedule, I'm sure your plan wouldn't be to eat a full roast turkey dinner with all the trimmings on that night, would it? As part of your overall plan it may be counted as a light bite night, something easy to prepare, wholesome, delicious, and light in nature reducing tiredness and enabling concentration. The evening class will be a distraction. You may plan to walk to and from the venue to add some movement into the mix along the way. Plan constantly and make sure nutritional intake is part of the plan.

As well as all suggestions being made positively to the unconscious mind, all suggestions need to be delivered with emotion. Great business or sports people talk about passion. They want this thing more than anything. It's not will power they are describing it's an emotion to succeed, a powerful feeling that when cognitively associated with the suggestions drives the meaning home. If you were to make a list of all the things that you wanted to achieve and then graded the list A to C, with A being the activity or goal that will give you the most and deepest satisfaction, it is clear to see which items in the list you will more easily achieve. This emotion is created and nurtured from the life around you, the people that you come into contact with, family, friends and colleagues. Why do you really want to lose weight? Is it to please your family, to set a good example to your children or to stem the misgivings recently issued by your doctor? All of these things have a deep seated connection to your emotions. If your reason for losing weight is because somebody at work looks better than you or you may want to look a bit better in your Christmas gown, the element of success will hardly return any level of emotion and more often than not, no increased satisfaction. If you continually set goals that when achieved create an overwhelming amount of pride and self fulfilment, you will create a heightened level of ability in all areas of your life. The life I am talking about is truly amazing.

Right at this moment, are you satisfied with life?

It may to all intents and purposes be a good and rewarding life, your role as part of the family unit, an important one, where others rely on your input and calming nature. But, on a personal level is this enough? What's in it for you? Being contented is a pattern, a routine that is delivering an outcome. Train tracks that have already formed, the habits that make you the way you are, the way you feel about yourself and the way you look. By changing the pattern of what we do, we can change the outcome of who we are and come rain or high water, we can feel more satisfaction and greater levels of self fulfilment.   Stay in one place for only so long, continue to plan and break the pattern, looking for better ways to do things. This overall attitude, of constant small improvement and change driven through every part of your life will focus the importance of a healthy balanced existence. If I asked you to take up dancing to lose weight it would work for a while. I'm sure you'd enjoy it, dancing is fun after all, but how long would it be before you'd slip into deep ruts again, held back by misgivings and lapses of purpose? Reinvent your life regularly. Try everything. Importantly create memories, tearful ones, hard earned ones, funny ones, the whole gambit. Bank them and create a montage of photographs. Don't leave them on a laptop hard drive or in a box, put them on display. Have a wacky wall somewhere, a graphical timeline of where you were and where you are now, leaving space for the future. Having sorted through thousands of photographs from the nineties, I had an impressive timeline of foreign travel, albeit represented by a rather uncomfortably overweight representation of my former self and I didn't like what I saw. When it came to the noughties I realised I had very little photographic evidence to show for my efforts, few documented memories. A decade in my case it seemed, ruled by a relentless workload solely for an employer's benefit. I must have done more with my life, but it was almost impossible to stake a claim to any major achievement. Pictures help you to appreciate what you've achieved, from milestones in your children's growth to days out at the beach or rewards for hard work, put them on display. Put them in a prominent place and listen for the comments from visitors to your home. Are you ahead? Are your children experiencing new things every week under your tutelage? An extraordinary life is down to you.

Creating the right mindset

The right mindset comes from using your imagination. A part of our cognitive make up that for most of us has lay dormant since our years of early learning. We traversed from a world of discovery in our school years, which nurtured our abilities to work outside of the box to a working world where barriers and rules dominate the landscape. We learn to conform, to fit in with our social environment and behave within acceptable boundaries. In mainstream terms, we start work at 9am and finish at 5pm, live for the freedom of the weekend and have more month than money. Only a few so called visionaries break the mould and become entrepreneurial.

Visionary is an interesting word. Visionary implies the creation of pictures, predominantly depicting a future, not in the past. A person that can see what they want, define its boundaries clearly and strive to achieve it.

How many visionaries have you heard of, that have failed along the way?

The answer is lots of them. In fact every successful business person can recall in graphic detail the road to success and the many setbacks that have needed to be overcome to achieve the ultimate goal. Some of these setbacks may be as serious as going bust and losing everything, before final resurrection into the land of the achiever. I am not saying put everything you own on the line, but successful business is a clear analogy with losing weight.   There is no doubt, on this journey there will be times that you simply cannot adhere to strict portion control and nutritional timetables life isn't like that, but the occasional blip does not make an overweight person.

Using visionary thinking is one of the big methods used in the therapy room to bring about positive change.   Imagine a mirror containing your reflection, not your image as you see it now, but the new you. Close your eyes and see that image exactly the way that you want to be, will be, in 6 or 12 months time. The picture will invoke feeling. You'll notice your physiology change. You'll sit back and smile more. Feeling lighter has an overall effect on your life. Now step inside the mirror and look around. Get up close and see the clothes that you are wearing, your stature, imagine the mirror image reflecting you in different situations. Having an interview, going to work, at a party, relaxing at home, all of these situations will have changed in subtle and definitive ways. Now turn around three hundred and sixty degrees and see how everything that interacts with you has also changed. Friends, family, colleagues, even people you don't already know will be playing a new role. As you change, so will the attitudes of the people around you, some will embrace your success and add to your motivation, where others will fail to understand that change is needed to bring the fulfilment you need. There are bright beams of light surrounding the things in your life that are exciting, refreshing and new. Now step out of the mirror and walk backwards slowly. There is a path directly in front of you leading to the mirror. The journey that you are now on takes you directly to the mirror where you and the new you will become one, all you have to do is take one step at a time.

Now it doesn't matter if you listen to this message on an audio file or just close your eyes and direct your own mind to accept this picture, you are choosing your own direction and destiny. This picture is your subconscious self image and is key to your success. If you keep a doubtful image in your mind, an overweight image you are never truly on the journey, merely a bystander waiting for it to happen. In fact those with an overweight image can expect to have two wardrobes of clothes, thin clothes and fat clothes to allow for both parts of the yo-yo cycle.

Alternative behaviours

To break out of the mould of normalised thinking, each behaviour we engage in needs to be scrutinised and being critical of our actions is harder than you think. The rules we have for behaviour that resides in our minds, our beliefs and values will be different for each of us, like a grey band of operating code constantly moving. We can only truly see this difference if we communicate with others. The world outside of our local awareness is vast and the more experience we have in communication, the greater our chances of appreciation and empathy.

With experience we can look at our own behaviours and decide to stay the same or change to better our situation. What are these behaviours? Well, in short everything we do or say is a behaviour. If we get out of bed at 8am every day, ask yourself why do I do this? Do I need that length of sleep? Am I up just in time for work? What do I do with the time between breakfast and work?

For some of us the answers may speak for themselves. Maybe there is just enough time to eat before making the dash to work in the rush hour. For others, 8am might mean the maximum amount of sleep before a foodless cycle to work. So what is the alternative behaviour? Could you exchange 15 minutes of sleep for a small walk each morning? After a healthy breakfast could you review your plan for the day, ensuring that you have all you need? Perhaps making notes and creating ideas.

The alternative behaviour doesn't need to be large, as I emphasised earlier lots of little changes when actioned together will break you out of the rut.   Constantly review, analyse and make small changes to your life. These changes offer long term weight loss management and lifestyle change. Maybe consider:

Why do I get an hour for lunch and I sit at my desk and surf the internet?

When I go to a party, am I the one sitting and not dancing?

What memory could I be creating right now, instead of sitting in a warm living room at the weekend?

What is my routine on a school night? Can I identify patterns that could so easily be broken?

After a meal, am I affected in anyway? Do these include tiredness, lethargy, negative feelings?

The patterns we continue to use become hard coded and difficult to change. For instance, you may have a job, you work hard, long hours, Monday to Friday and you deserve to relax at the weekend. Your downtime includes good food, treats out, cakes from the delicatessen and a well deserved take away. You deserve it right, or what is the point of going to work. When you've achieved stability in life, marriage, children, the patterns are easier to identify and seemingly harder to change. Remember balance is what you are trying to achieve. Yes you deserve treats, a nice chocolate latte and a slice of cake and even a stuffed crust pizza, but no one ever created a great memory in a coffee shop. How many people do you know get their camera phone out and take a snap of their family whilst eating carrot cake, not many and even less people would want to see the picture.

Turn this thing on its head. The weekend is approaching. You have four or five of them in a month. You have a family, a partner or friends, it is down to you as the alpha male/female to set the goal, chuck in a selection of ideas and motivate the creation of memories. Don't get me wrong a trip to a theme park is a wonderful day out, but not within everybody's realm of affordability. Whatever you set out to do doesn't have to cost a lot of money, albeit some travelling expense and a packed lunch. The UK is a treasure trove of attraction from country parks, churches, hills and mountains, zoos, monuments that few countries can rival. Use the internet and search the local area first and create a list of things that appeal to you. Each place may be as small as a thirty minute visit or a full day trip. It all depends on how you want to fit it in. An iron-age hill fort in the pouring rain may not appeal to all but the hardy walker and from time to time you will get it wrong, not every attraction will motivate your entourage. But these are the memories that you will remember. When you made the effort and something went wrong or you got soaking wet or the car broke down, although miserable at the time these memories will make you laugh in the future. But Steve, what the hell has this got to do with weight loss?

The whole time you are moving, motivating you are creating emotion. Park the car and walk and enjoy, laugh create more of the pleasure energy. Take a packed lunch with you, perhaps a cool box or back-pack of food to share. It doesn't have to be boring sandwiches, change the food for each occasion. Food for a day at point to point horse racing should match the occasion or if you are taking on the mighty Snowden, you may require more than a cheese sandwich and an energy bar.

On reflection you've been out on a Saturday saw a few interesting things, took a few photographs and used up valuable relaxation time, how are you going to be feeling on Monday morning? Are you scared that your next week at work will be more tiring? That you might be too tired to make it through the week?

Fast forward to Monday morning and you hear the usual question. "How was your weekend?"

What will your answer be? "Fantastic!"

Your answer will exude all of the pleasure energy as opposed to "the usual, didn't do much and oh, it's Monday morning." How long will it take before people around you begin to see the change in you? Just something a little bit different, something they won't be able to put their finger on.   The world is rampaged by stress and depression. More people are taking anti-depressants than ever before, we all need that pick up and why not you.   Take the lead. The patterns you control are all important.

Adding direction to your nutritional intake - high quality, small amounts

Your body deserves fine dining. A pattern has developed inside you that accepts a colossal amount of poor quality food be consumed in record breaking times. We shovel down our meals at high velocity with the bulk of the food going directly to our stomachs, missing our taste buds. We do not feel full until the entire meal has found its final resting place in the base of our stomach, then it's too late to do anything about it. The brain receives the signal, you are full and it really is too late, your plate is empty. At best the feeling of being full is a discomfort followed by tiredness and lethargy, at worst painful cramps often accompany guilt perpetuating the yo-yo diet cycle even further. Along with guilt comes regret, the internal vocalisation ringing in your ears, "never again", but the feeling doesn't last long. Within an hour you can feel well enough to continue on, stuffing your face with savouries and all possible concoction of idling product.

That's what we do now. The way forward is to plan. If you know in advance what you are going to eat, the ingredients have all been sourced in advance and you can prepare the finished dish in a reasonable amount of time you lessen the issue of choosing the old food types. When you place the items on the plate, stop and take a moment. Think about design. Even if you are eating on your own, place the cooked ingredients on the plate with some thought and sincerity. Piling up mashed potato is hardly ever going to look good, but placing it within a steel ring not only reduces the amount of carbohydrate you eat, it offers a suitable platform for the protein to reside. No matter what size of plate you use create a design that you can see more of the plate than the food. It now looks appetising.

Set the table with the minimum of a placemat, seasoning and cutlery. Turn off all distractions, your phone, the TV and the internet or newspaper. Taste each part of the meal, the protein, the carbohydrate and the vegetables in turn and really taste them. What are your culinary skills really like? Have you done justice to this quality produce?

Now major on this new pattern, tasting the food. Eat the food slowly, chewing each small fork of produce, letting your mouth empty before divulging in the next portion. Placing your knife and fork down and entering into conversation will give you sufficient time for digestion. What we are doing here is making the whole occasion special. The pattern you are creating is creating a discerning palate. You will soon discover that not all that you prepare is good enough to eat. By eating a little at a time it becomes almost impossible to continue eating something that doesn't meet your exacting standards. As the food disappears become aware that your stomach will begin to sense when enough is enough, read those signals and don't overeat. Less is always more.

At the end of the meal sit for a few moments and allow the last remnants to pass into digestion and let your brain identify how you feel. It may take a few meals at first to create the correct associations, but you should always feel as if you could eat more. This is a pleasure feeling, not a pain. Complete enjoyment is when the food suits your palate, the taste is high quality and imaginative and you don't have the feeling of being bloated.

Create alternative behaviours when you know you are going to be vulnerable

Outside of the prescribed meal zone, temptation is all around. We have identified these in our patterns. An alternative behaviour is an antidote. If putting the kids to bed at 8pm allows you time to relax and divulge in extracurricular feeding activities, then it is time to break the pattern. Find something else to do. Quiet time is not only a time to relax, but a time to achieve. By planning you will need pockets of time to decide on new recipes, create buying lists of ingredients and research new and exciting activities. By losing weight and being more energetic you will need less down time. In fact when the pleasure energy is flowing, making the body move will be preferable to quiet sedation.

The box of tricks in the corner of our living rooms, the kitchen and bedrooms has a lot to do with creating the wrong type of patterns. The TV delivers a set piece of not-to-miss episodes strung out seemingly haphazardly throughout your schedule. One series ending as another begins, the run up to Christmas with Strictly Come Dancing and X-Factor vying for your already stretched time. The TV is both inspirational and detrimental in our lives. We can see so many examples of the world around us in every episode, yet we choose to watch more than we choose to do. The TV offers variety. With so many channels it is hard to not find something that satisfies our wants and needs. But, and there is a but. We only have a finite amount of time and something has to give.   On those cold nights in the winter it is hard to imagine doing anything else than snuggling up in front of the fire with a good movie, but is the opposite true in the summer months.

Is your TV turned on regardless of your requirements?

Is your life soap centric?

With digital recording as simple as it is now, do we need to comply with the patterns laid down by the independent channels or the BBC's view of reality. I return to our old friend planning. When you create a plan that works towards your defined goals, prime time will need to be identified. For instance, your goals may be to include exercise in your daily routine, to enjoy creating prose in the form of poetry and a little time to develop your understanding of the classic French recipes. Now when we do this, won't necessarily be the same for all of us. The prime time in a person's life will often be different for a person on nights, a mother with children or someone working within the bounds of a nine to five schedule. When planning to achieve, allocate the main activity into your prime time slot for the day. It might be a two hour period in mid evening or three half hour periods of calm in your day, it's up to you. Identify them and say to yourself I am going to achieve this thing at that time. It is amazing what you can achieve in thirty minutes if you set your mind to it. What was the alternative, feet up, decent coffee, a biscuit treat and yet more unplanned TV?

The whole point of what I profess is, make small, regular, changes and you won't even notice the difference, but you will feel the impact. By simply applying yourself for four half hours per week, you will have focussed for 8-10 hours a month. You can do a whole lot of interesting stuff in a month. I wrote my first novel in four years around a very business orientated work life schedule. I was never tempted to get down to typing a few hundred words at lunch, how ridiculous. I had a limiting belief that I could not do anything constructive unless I settled down in the total silence of my office. Nowadays, I've broken that pattern. I write to a plan using small spare moments in the day. On top of all my other achievements in the year my literary works appear using time I would have previously squandered. I don't suffer in anyway, I don't need a chocolate biscuit and I don't think about food in that time, due to the distraction of the text. I could of course, have allocated this time to stick my coat on and walk around the block. Remember ½ a mile of physical exercise is not the end of the earth, you don't need to change into gym kit and you certainly won't need a packed lunch to make it happen. Balance must come into play. The planning phase will be heavily influenced by what you like doing the most. If you are overweight, exercise will have always come second in your thinking, well now it comes first. If you have thirty minutes, three times a day of prime time, make two of those sessions of movement. Pleasure will repay you with clarity and positive thought energy with the remaining 30 minutes.

Chapter 3 - Planning your Future

The plan – turn your life into a business

Before we begin to plan our approach we may want to consider and assess your balance wheel.   The balance wheel contains a series of segments which indicate the satisfaction you attach to your areas of life. We are only truly in balance when the wheel runs perfectly smoothly. It is unusual however, for us to be content in all areas of our lives but it does show where we need to focus.

*The Balance Wheel is taken from Coaching with NLP by Joseph O'Connor and Andrea Lages.

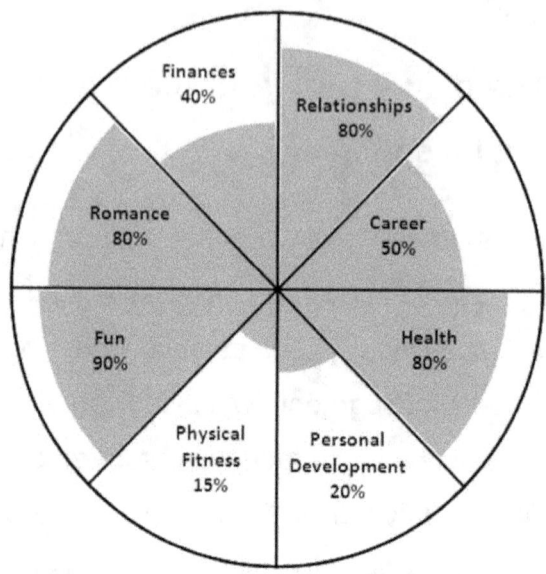

Finances
40%

Relationships
80%

Romance
80%

Career
50%

Fun
90%

Health
80%

Physical
Fitness
15%

Personal
Development
20%

When you look at the segments of the wheel you need to be truthful to yourself. Grade your own experience of each section. Give yourself a score of 1, if you are completely dissatisfied with the particular area of your life and a 10, if completely satisfied. The height of your score in each segment is unimportant on its own, it is only when we begin to compare it with the rest of the wheel can we truly acknowledge where we need to change.

Take a moment to consider if the wheel shows a lack of satisfaction in health & fitness and wealth, how will this affect your decisions in where to set goals?

Rarely will anyone achieve complete satisfaction. In fact, those people that are happy with their lot may need to look a little deeper and with more clarity.   You are reading a weight loss book aren't you? Is being completely satisfied with your life, giving you the figure you've always desired or have you got the ability to reach a little higher?   Achievement in any of these areas will always promote self confidence and purpose, continue to build, adapt and stretch your own possibilities.

Know what you want - set goals

In exactly the same way as a successful business executive will project their vision of where they want to be in five, ten or fifteen years time, so must you. Depending on where you are in your life right now, may alter the time periods in which you want to achieve, but everything else is the same. A teenager has the opportunity to race ahead and visualise success right into retirement. Whereas, those of us that have already seen some of life may be planning for shorter periods, even looking to exceed normal retirement dates or generate enough income to create security. The importance of building a picture of exactly what you want is vital. I say picture, but this is not the only one of your senses you should employ. When you close your eyes and use your imagination build pictures with sounds, feelings, tastes and smells. Make these images as strong as you can. Now write them down. Write down you goals and be specific. Goals can be segmented into long, medium and short term. The short term, immediate things that you want to experience now, plays at the theatre, places that you want to visit, etc. The medium term is for those things that cost a little more, dream holidays, qualifications that will help you move towards your longer term aims and more. Things that fall into the long term are pension planning, where you would ultimately like to live, the security and wellbeing of your family. I once heard the entrepreneurial guru Tony Robbins describe this process of chunking as a way of taking the larger dreams and breaking them down into seemingly easily achievable elements. This is absolutely correct. You won't go from fat to thin in a moment. If you move towards your dream weight as part of a total lifestyle choice, there is no doubt your self esteem will soar.

How do I set my dreams and goals?

Use your imagination. One of the promises of hypnosis is that your imagination is expanded way beyond your wildest dreams. Without imagination you will never break out of the rut, the pattern that is holding you back. Go mad. You don't have to show the list to anybody. Write it down quickly without conscious thought. If you take too much time your critical thinking will get in the way and start asking all sorts of internal questions that will kill the process. Be spontaneous, off the wall. Be as daft as you like – write! If you want to go to the moon, write it down. The subconscious mind automatically processes thoughts without question as a long as they are within the realms of possibility. So, why not write them down. If you've wanted to be a train driver or a ballet dancer since you were young, write it down. If we begin to dream the creative juices will begin to create pathways in your subconscious mind. Will you have lost anything if you finally drive a train at a museum or watch a ballet on the stage? Of course not, but you have created memories that you otherwise wouldn't have achieved.

When you create the list, continue with it. Don't just put it in a draw and forget about it. Keep it close by and add and improve as often as you can. Find a way of making notes all the time. How many times have you dreamed something in your sleep and can't remember it in the morning? Get a small pad with a pen or a folded sheet of A4, put it in your hand bag or back pocket. I know a lot of people will prefer the iPhone approach with a carefully crafted app that allows for note taking and filtering. If that floats your boat then go for it, but it isn't necessary to make it happen. By committing words to paper you are actively setting the imagination in motion, reaffirming the message in the conscious mind and beginning the process of achievement. By activating the imagination the thought is already bypassing your critical thinking and moving into the subconscious zone. In actual fact, you are already starting to move towards the goal that you've written. Having all of your goals written in one place means that you can speed up their progression.

Activating the plan

In front of you is a list of the things you feel passionate about. Are you sure? Is everything on the list something that will really create emotion and memories? Think about it. If you have a list of things that are less than inspiring on some level, how will you ever find the motivation to achieve them?

Have you been specific? I would like to climb Snowdon someday or I would like to pass my motorcycle test is not specific, is it? Open ended goals will always get achieved, someday. I would like to be four stone lighter, some day. If climbing a mountain is your dream, then why not this summer, in June. The weather will be good for walking and now with a period in mind you can make the arrangements for accommodation, gathering the right equipment and book the holiday from work. Planning for weight loss is straight forward. For most of us, aiming to lose 1and ½ lbs per week is achievable and sustainable. With this amount in mind, you can clearly calculate what weight you will be at given dates in your diary. Taking this as an example, you could say with three months (13 weeks) to Christmas, I will be 19.5lbs lighter (1.4 stones), followed by a further 19.5lbs at Easter and so on. Within this short period of time and almost three stones in weight lighter, the benefits in the way you feel, your health and energy levels will all have soared.

When you write down the goal give it a clear title, such as Summer Holiday Weight Loss or My First 10k Run. The title should always have a meaning. Below the title, explain your desired outcome, again give reasons and be expressive. Give two clear paragraphs about your desired outcome.

Summer Holiday Weight Loss

For my holiday in Cyprus leaving on the 27th of July, 2015, I will be 11 stone, 9 pounds. This weight loss of two stones, 6 pounds is possible by losing 1 and ½ pounds per week. I am committed to exercise and will walk a mile each morning before work, increasing this activity in the evenings on at least three occasions each week.

By planning weekly meals I will add one additional new recipe to my culinary repertoire and eliminate take away food in this period. The additional exercise will increase my energy levels which will be allocated to at least four hours of quality time at the weekend, visiting interesting places or playing sport.

When you write down the date, the time, the weight, the number of times you intend to do the thing or a time over the finishing line, whatever you decide is right for you, write it down and be precise.   If your goal is to run a road race, remember the fundamentals of the pleasure and pain principle. It is good to run to aid weight loss. However it is not a good idea to run on the road for extended periods if you are carrying excessive weight. Pardon the pun. Learn to walk before you can run. A commitment you can make is to book your place ahead of time. Put the date in your diary and build up appropriately. In terms of beginners times these can be recorded during training and used to measure progress. Prior to the race set a time over the line.   There is lots of advice on running on the internet with preset plans available for every form of training. I did say for some of you, your eyes would glaze over at this point. Goals of this magnitude take long term commitment, you will get there.

So let's recap. You now know what you want to achieve, you are being specific about when it's going to happen and now you need to oil the wheels of achievement and plan each specific task to get you to where you need to be. Every time you sit and spend time looking at this subject, ask the question of yourself 'what can I do right now that will advance my progress?' Too many of us buy self help programs and give up before we read them. Some plan and plan and plan and take no action using every excuse under the sun. You are not that person, you will take action. In my early days of writing I spent three months working out the storyline on large white boards before transferring it to word document. Within two weeks of beginning to write, the whole story had taken a detour and much of the material had not been used. I wasted too much time on thinking, not doing. You see, creative juices flow at every moment on your journey, your good ideas will be superseded or upgraded because you are using your imagination. I guarantee you will achieve 90% of your first list within months. Do something now. If you have aspirations to be an author or an artist, do something now. A few words or a new technique, expose your mind to something new, right now. We are still talking about weight loss, right? You bet we are. You can bet on one thing, right in front of you is a plan. A plan of the new you. An exciting new person who moves, who acts, who seeks out exciting things to eat and puts their health first.

Plan to rest

Read this statement two or three times, make sure my explanation of rest and relaxation is exactly the same as your understanding. Sitting with your feet up, watching a TV soap with a chocolate bar and a glass of wine is not relaxing. Having an extra three hours in bed on a Sunday morning is not relaxation. Both of these things may feel amazing. After a long week at work I'm sure you'll feel like those few extra moments a real luxury. These are the activities that you associate with feeling good now. The more luxurious parts of your life and you yearn for more of these. Even successful business people focus everything on making it big and when they get enough time to do more of this stuff they soon become bored and many return to work in one way or another. Challenge your current accepted thinking. We do need to de-stress and we do need to get an acceptable amount of regular sleep these are imperative to achieve this long list of goals that we have now identified. I've mentioned before that true relaxation is reduction of activity in the conscious and unconscious minds, essentially switching them to tick over mode. So that no thoughts are rattling around, distracting you. You may think that watching the TV is relaxing, but it isn't. At another level you continue to process the thoughts of the day. Incidents in the office, problems with the children and disagreements with your spouse all come to the front of your thinking as you stop other less important thoughts being processed. The detrimental pressures of life that have plagued you in the day overwhelm your subconscious mind as it tries to bring resolution or answers. These thoughts become dominant. After the TV you go to bed and the conscious mind takes a back seat while the subconscious seeks to protect and put accepting thoughts into action. A mind full of stressful thoughts a good night sleep does not make. In fact in the morning you feel like you haven't slept at all. In retrospect, lying in bed later at the weekend diminishes the amount of time you have to enjoy free time and offers yet further opportunity for your critical thinking to get in the way. A Sunday may also generate the back to work on Monday syndrome, where you feel your whole life is about work and the weekend is over before it's started.

Find thirty minutes a day to relax. Meditation and self hypnosis are skills that can be learned and when practised offer dramatic effect's few others will ever realise. This first step in relaxation will put you immediately light years ahead of your friends and colleagues developing an open and active mind, clarity of thought, less tiredness and more energy and a greater ability at focus on what's important.

What is self hypnosis?

Some say that, all hypnosis is self hypnosis. The hypnotic process is a series of linked instructions that guide your thinking, almost like taking a journey from start to end. Self hypnosis can be achieved in a number of ways with either a recorded message or by exploring the techniques a hypnotherapist uses to create self guidance. Both methods can be found in all manner of sports preparation, producing a focussed and positive mindset to complement already heightened skills in the chosen activity. In comparison a hypnotherapist delivers instruction, whilst identifying key physiological change in the subject. The process of hypnosis as described by artful hypnotist Igor Ledochowski is that hypnosis occurs in three main phases or the ABS formula.   A. Have the full attention of the hypnotee.   B. Bypass the critical thinking of the conscious mind and S. stimulate the unconscious mind with the information and mindset of your prescribed goals.

So many things can be achieved by the self discipline of hypnosis. At first the benefits of true relaxation are realised, then with practise and focussing on your goals and ambitions means that you have clear direction to allow these things to happen. There are so many people that use these techniques before any major event in their lives, sportsmen get in the zone, essentially putting them, in a place where the world around them is turned off and the focus is directed at the finishing line. Racing drivers sit in the car on the line and imagine the circuit, the corners the gears, a mental practise. I have even spent time with people so crippled and debilitated with pain that they can represent the feeling of pain to the brain in a new way and live more comfortably. Self hypnosis has worked for hundreds of years and the only thing that is stopping you is the

time that you put into yourself and your
achievements.

Goals have hardly anything to do with losing weight

It's true.   Not all of your goals are going to be directly linked to weight loss. But indirectly, these goals are the most important aspect of your life and make sustained weight loss possible. For the obese in our society, weight and food are the two things that dominate their existence. No hour goes by without the thought of what's next, followed by the accompanying guilt or shame, components of the yo-yo diet. Few people in this area have any other outlook. The emotion felt is often enough to debilitate them socially, slowly removing them from activities in society that they would otherwise be included. The effects of social and physical withdrawal are normally slow and undetectable. So slow that the person is rarely able to identify the changes albeit the cumulative effect of additional weight. Now I can't say that all overweight people are sad, some have a persona that throws them back into the mix with gregariousness and confidence. What lies beneath the surface can only be surmised. Some accept their size and get on with life others battle continuously in the background trying each fad diet as it comes along, always with the same result.   It is difficult to compare two people who sit confidently in the world, the overweight person with a public persona or the athletic individual who has established euphoria by exercise and healthy living. You may look beyond the mask of happiness in the overweight and believe that their world of exercise and nutrition is not in balance and therefore positivity could be a facade to protect the way they are viewed by others. When a person transforms their shape and mindset the energy is true with a pureness that radiates positivity, an energy that congruently reflects their mental well being.

Before planning commences

   With food it is important to have some sort of record of what you are doing now to compare with the plan. If you make a note of what you eat, the results are always surprising. Keep the sheet in the kitchen, record every last molecule. You know by now that you don't need to feel guilty about what you have eaten so write it down. Be honest, record the date and the part of the day.   Breakfast, morning, lunch, dinner, evening etc. This information will help you to quickly identify the danger zones, when it is so easy to binge. In a couple of short weeks you'll know what you're up against. Which foods are the problems ones and at which time of the day are you most vulnerable.

How to plan activities for short, medium and long term

Get a diary or a sheet that shows a page a week. I know we are in the age of the iPhone and you'll want to run this operation like any other app, but in the first instance do it the old fashioned way with a pen and a piece of paper. The same diary pages can be used for both the nutritional and exercise elements of your plan. Remember whatever you decide to put in your plan it needs to balance. Taking one night a week to attend night school will be an opportunity to substitute an evening meal for a light bite or a day out walking at the weekend replacing a Sunday lunch with alternative pack up.

There is no need for me to lay the law down here stating the obvious facts that have been drilled into you on previous diets. Plenty of books on nutrition will give you this information and most of it is pretty useful.

Let's face it creating a habit of five pieces of vegetable and fruit a day is great thing to do. Never skip breakfast, reduce repetition in your meal schedules and include more of the healthy option are all great notions.

Let's get down to it, some short term goal planning. How long is short term? The answer is two to four weeks. Look at your list of goals and things you want to achieve. Local attractions and places of interest for instance, pick at least one to visit each weekend, block out an amount of time with travelling either side. Are you going on your own or with others, ring them now, firm up the appointment. Always be in control and ring again a few days before. This is as important as that big business deal, do everything you can to make it happen. On that day, what will be the eating arrangements? Maybe a packed lunch, returning to a light evening meal, I mean you won't to cook if you've been out for the day. Use your imagination something that takes ten minutes or less to prepare. Beans on toast, maybe a little obvious but Prawn cocktail can easily be elevated to a special offering. I am not here to dictate what you like or the benefits of its nutritional make up, this meal will be on the whole lighter. If the trip was a Saturday, then on the Sunday the meal may reflect the type of day. Perhaps local exercise near home, a country park or walk and a meal that needed thought in preparation. You have the time to try out a new recipe, to add it to the plate with care and attention and eat it slowly appreciating your work.

By getting the planning underway you can immediately see what produce you are going to need for the week ahead and buy from a list accordingly. I can promise you, buying from a list of ingredients will increase the quality of the products in your store room and reduce costs. The cost of food reduces because you will not tend to add the extras during the shop and eliminate the need to hold pre-prepared meals and frozen food. Eat fresh where possible. Remember your own restaurant may not have three Michelin stars yet, but your approach will have certainly turned the corner from a kitchen nightmare to professional purchasing.

Turning on the real life aspects

Each person's life will be unique to them. If you have teenagers for instance, the inevitable ferrying of children from one location to another can have an immediate impact on your planning. You may have the added pressure of creating different food groups for each age range in your family.

All you can do is your best. Sometimes it will work and other times it won't, don't beat yourself up. At the start, the things that are the hardest to change leave them alone and concentrate on something that you can action without much thought. You will find that as you gain momentum these more difficult areas will begin to change all by themselves.

Summary

Your life is your own and only you can and will want to alter its direction. When previously on a diet others may maliciously try to change your way of thinking by marginalising the decision you had made to change. Face the facts diets don't work and its easy for your will power to be disrupted. The Hypnotic Wisdom of Weight Loss is not will power and is not short term. By exercising the methods in this book you are creating a plan for an exceptional life, a lifestyle change that will create memories whichever way you turn giving you greater fulfilment. You will smile more. You'll have more friends and a whole new outlook. I still haven't mentioned weight loss have I? Your weight is just one element or your lifecycle, by setting goals and taking action you will move more. By planning what and when, you are already making tiny changes increasing the balance of healthiness. By feeling better and creating lots of that pleasure energy you cannot fail to succeed.